I0605371

TEEN GUIDE TO MENTAL HEALTH

TEEN GUIDE:
OBSESSIVE COMPULSIVE DISORDER

by Diana Murrell

BrightPoint Press

San Diego, CA

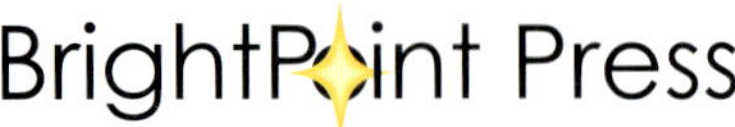

For more information, contact:
BrightPoint Press
PO Box 27779
San Diego, CA 92198
www.BrightPointPress.com

Content Consultant: Michelle Rozenman, PhD, assistant professor in the Department of Psychology, University of Denver

LIBRARY OF CONGRESS CATALOGING-IN-PUBLICATION DATA

Library of Congress Cataloging-in-Publication Data
Name: Murrell, Diana, author.
Title: Teen guide: obsessive compulsive disorder / by Diana Murrell.
Description: San Diego, CA: ReferencePoint Press, 2026 | Series: Teen guide to mental health | Audience: Grade 7 to 9 | Includes bibliographical references and index.
Identifiers: ISBN: 9781678211462 (hardcover) | ISBN: 9781678211479 (eBook)
The complete Library of Congress record is available at www.loc.gov.

CONTENTS

AT A GLANCE

- Obsessive compulsive disorder (OCD) is a mental health condition. People with OCD try to relieve themselves of distress caused by unwanted thoughts.

- Obsessions are unwanted and worrying thoughts. People can have obsessions about almost anything.

- Compulsions are actions that people with OCD do to feel better. Common compulsions include cleaning, asking for reassurance, and counting things.

- OCD does not have one simple cause. Instead, scientists have found several factors that may make OCD more likely to develop for some people than others.

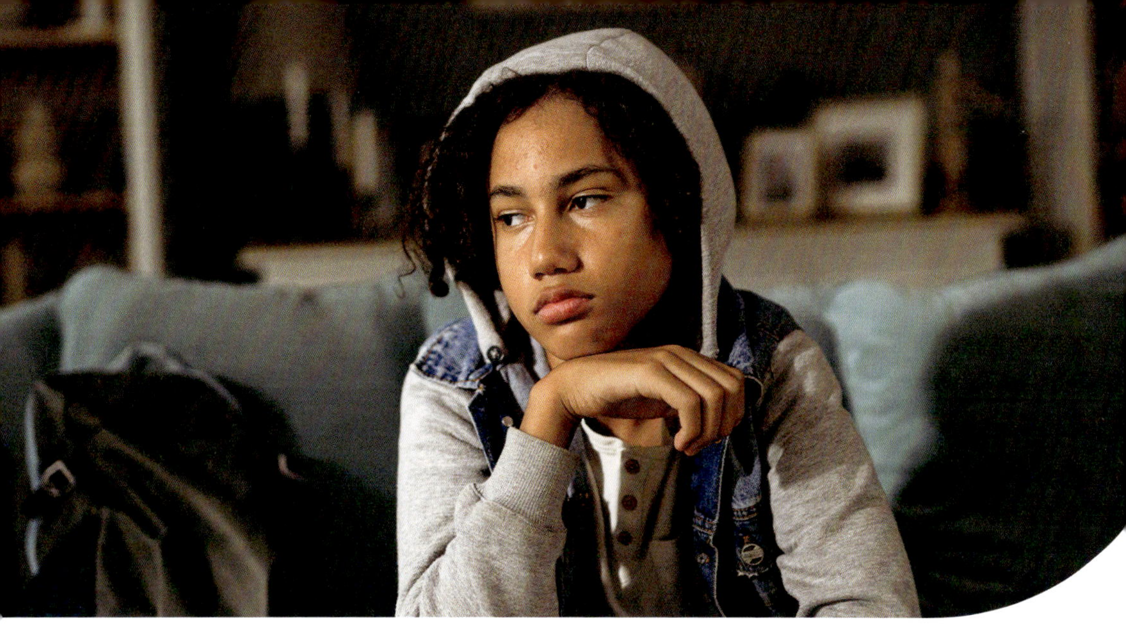

- OCD can affect a teen's daily life in many ways. It can take time and energy away from their education and their relationships with other people.

- The two main treatments for OCD are therapy and medication.

- The most effective form of therapy for OCD is exposure and response prevention (ERP). This treatment involves slowly and safely exposing a person with OCD to their fears with the support of a trained provider and with the patient's consent.

SUDDEN SCARY THOUGHTS

For as long as she could remember, Ivy had thoughts that disturbed her. She worried about accidentally stealing things. She confessed to her parents every little mistake she made. New thoughts began to bother her as a teenager. She feared that she unknowingly hurt people in her sleep. And she worried that she would forget to check whether her cat was sitting in the

Checking and rechecking potential sources of danger can sometimes be a symptom of OCD.

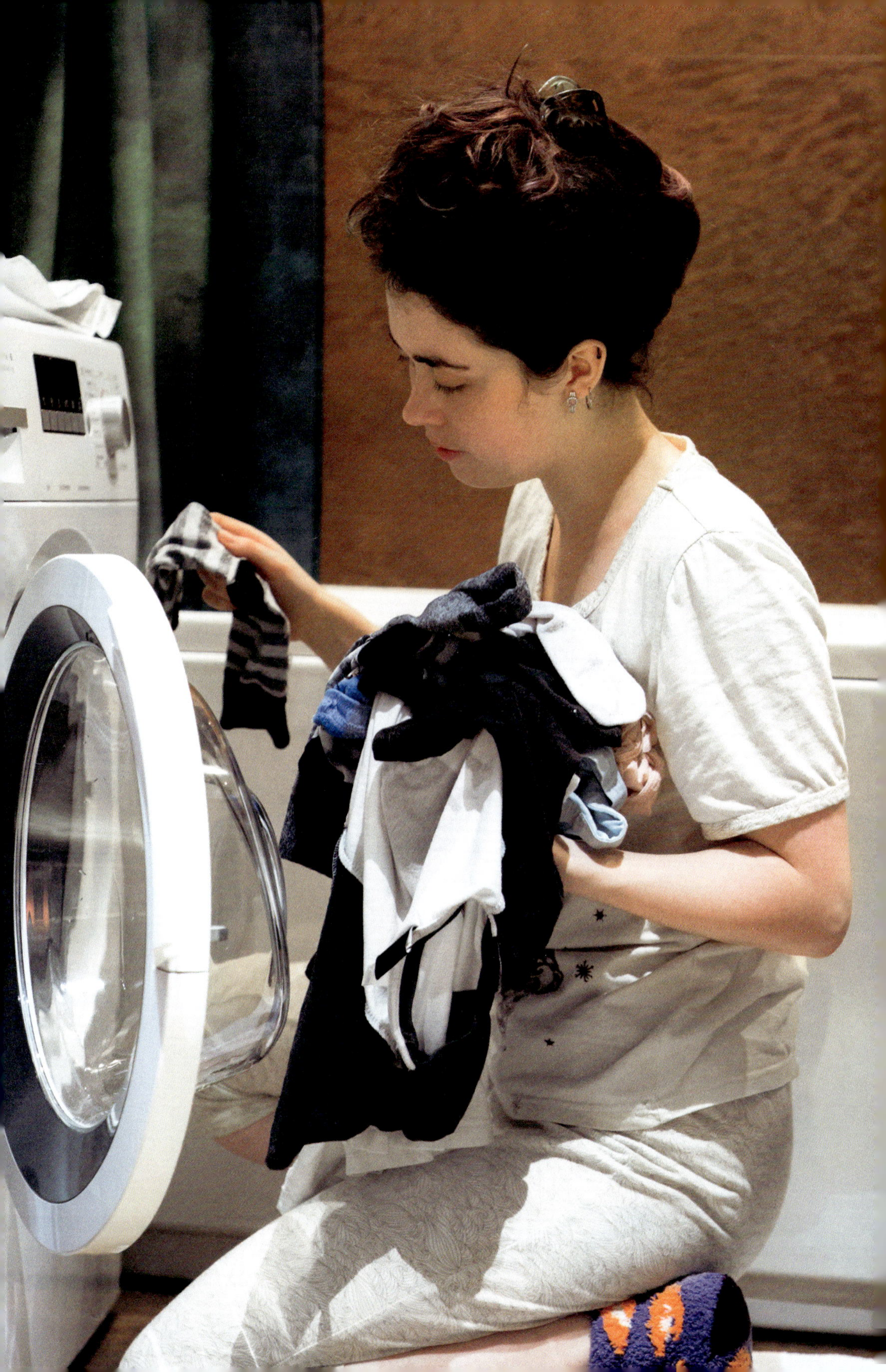

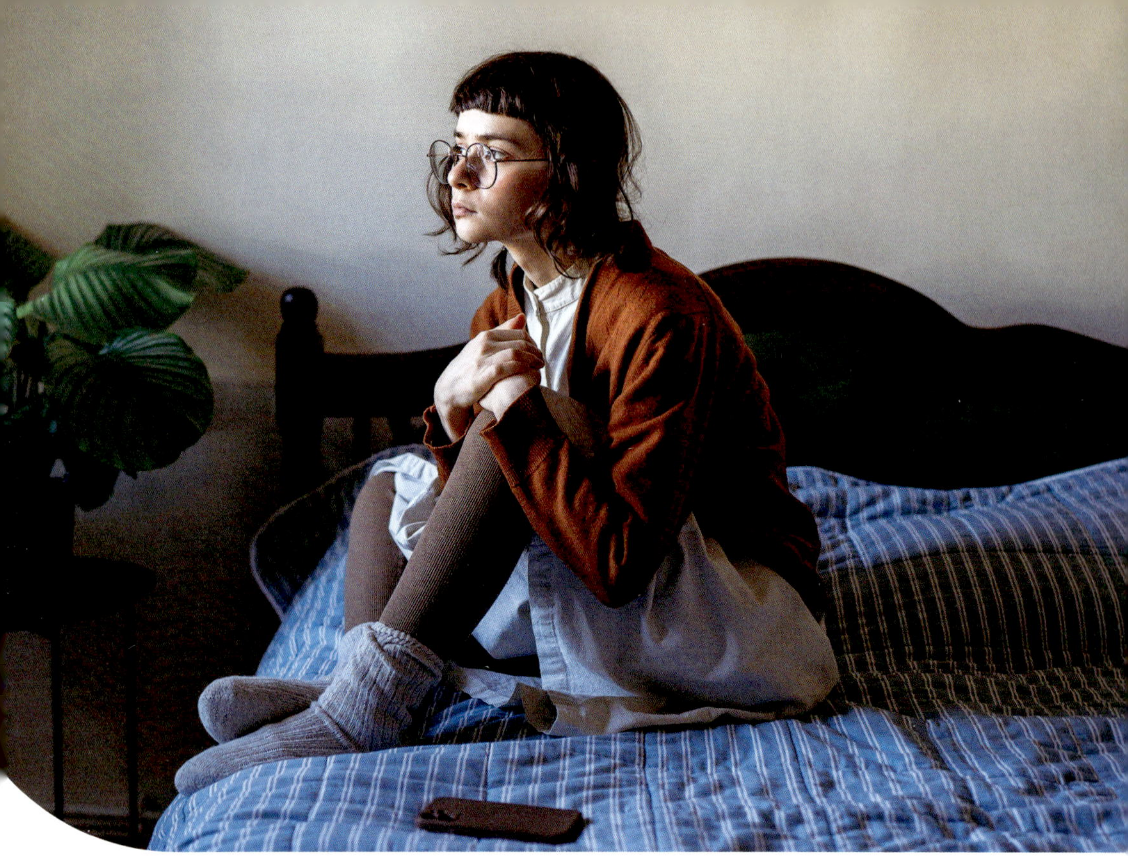

OCD can make a teen feel isolated from their loved ones.

dryer before starting it. She checked over and over again before starting the machine.

These negative thoughts and feelings made Ivy quiet around other people. She did not speak up much in school. Once, she skipped school entirely. The negative feelings slowly took over her life. She asked her family for help.

That was how Ivy learned that she had obsessive compulsive disorder (OCD). This mental health condition was causing her disturbing thoughts and feelings. She went to a treatment facility to see an OCD specialist. The specialist gave her treatments that helped her manage

OCD specialists are trained to provide evidence-based treatment for OCD.

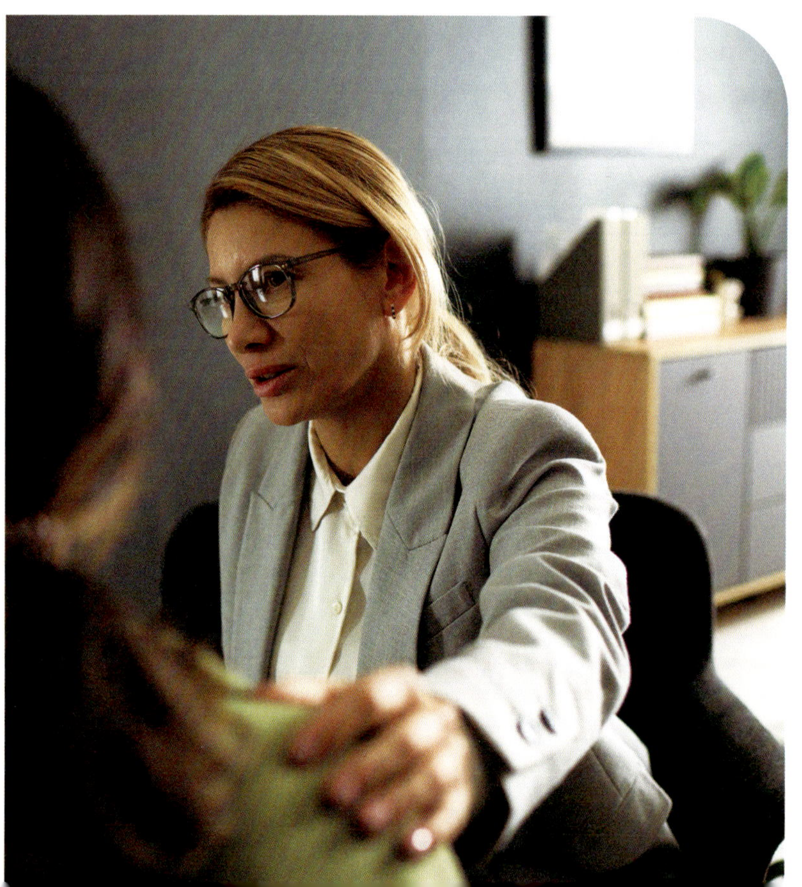

the condition. Ivy still manages her OCD today. She knows that there is no easy cure. But treatment allows her to take greater control of her life.

Many teens with OCD have success with specialized OCD treatments.

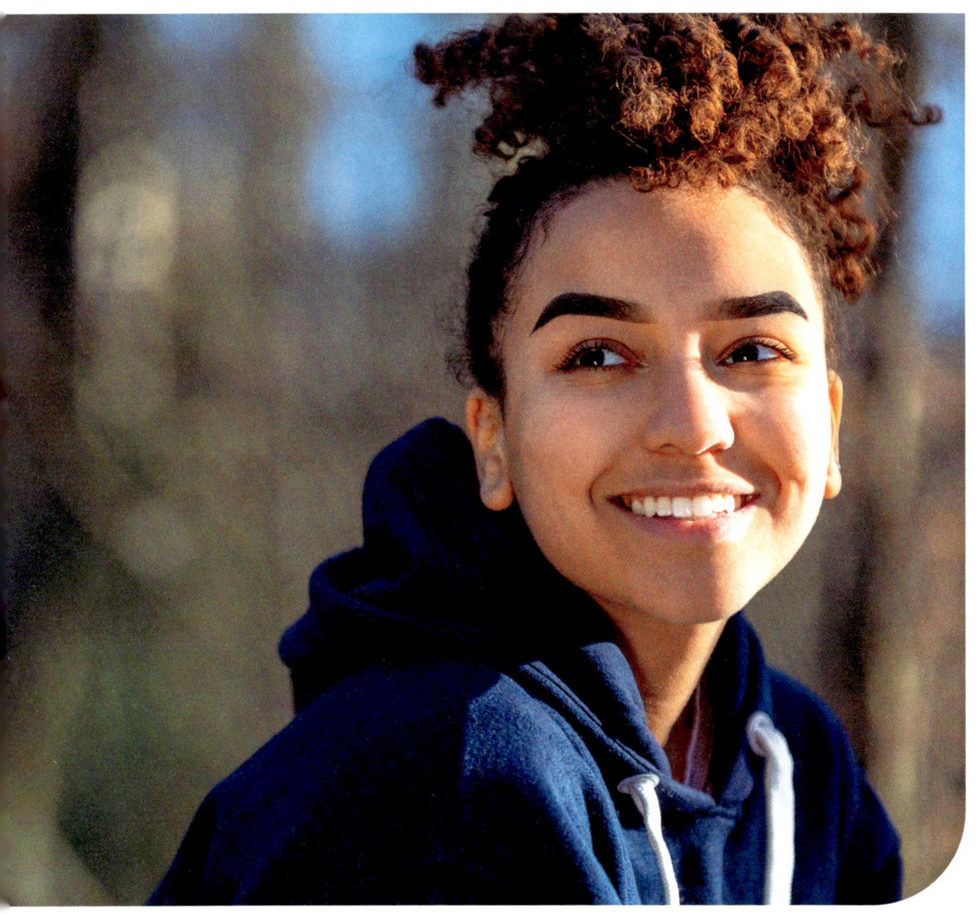

UNDERSTANDING OCD

Some people incorrectly think OCD simply means liking things clean and tidy. But it is more than that. OCD is a mental health condition. People with OCD have thoughts that upset them. They have trouble dismissing these thoughts. They do things to try to feel better. But it never feels like enough.

Treatments for OCD can help teens break this cycle. People with OCD can benefit from therapy. Sometimes **medication** can be helpful as well. These treatments can improve OCD symptoms. Over time, treatment can help teens with OCD feel better and accomplish their goals.

CHAPTER ONE

WHAT IS OCD?

OCD has two main parts. They are obsessions and compulsions. Obsessions are unwanted thoughts that cannot be controlled. They can be upsetting and scary. This distress leads people with OCD to engage in compulsions. Compulsions are behaviors people with OCD do or things they tell themselves to feel better.

OCD-related obsessions can be disturbing and overwhelming.

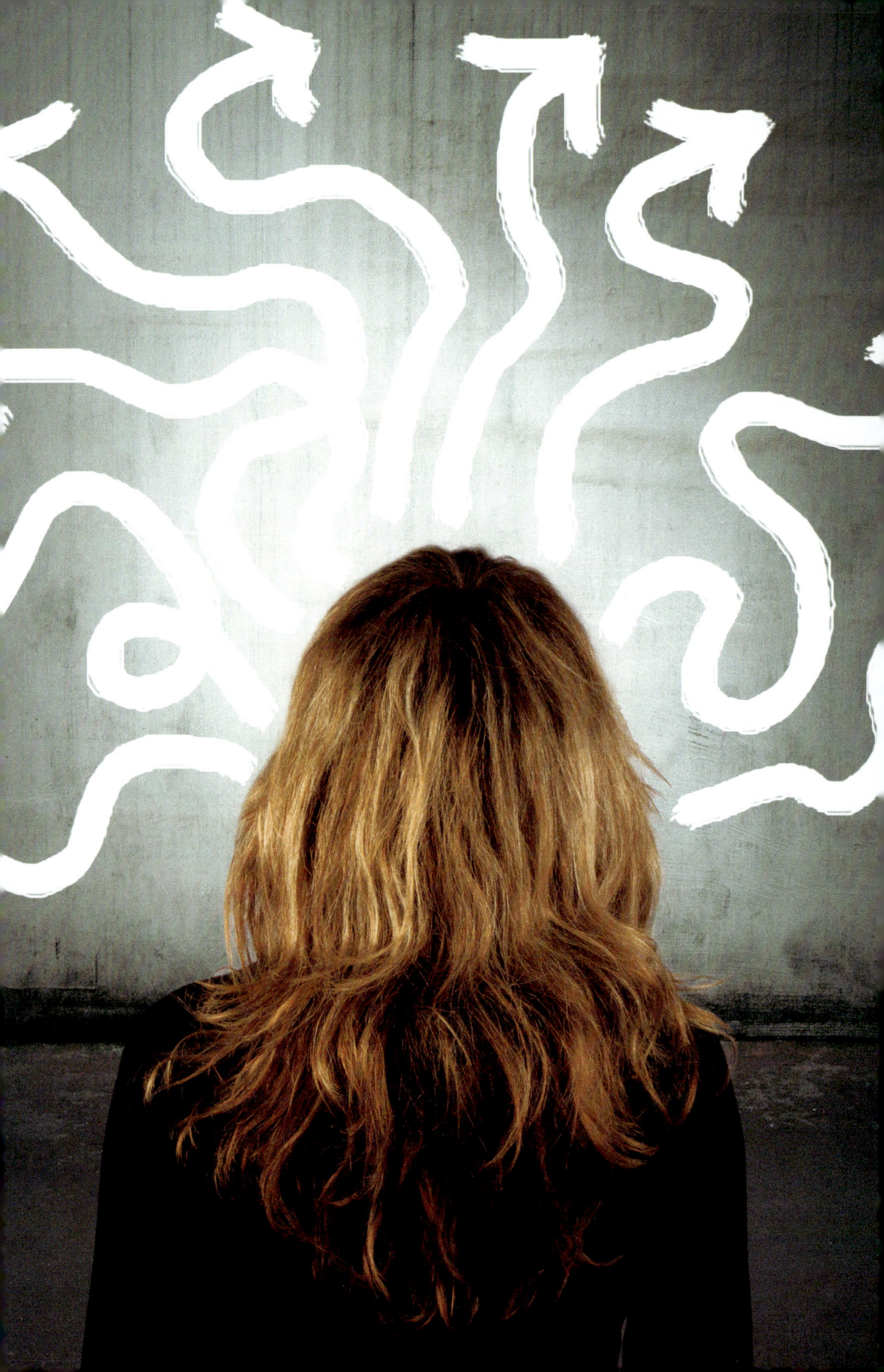

THE OCD CYCLE

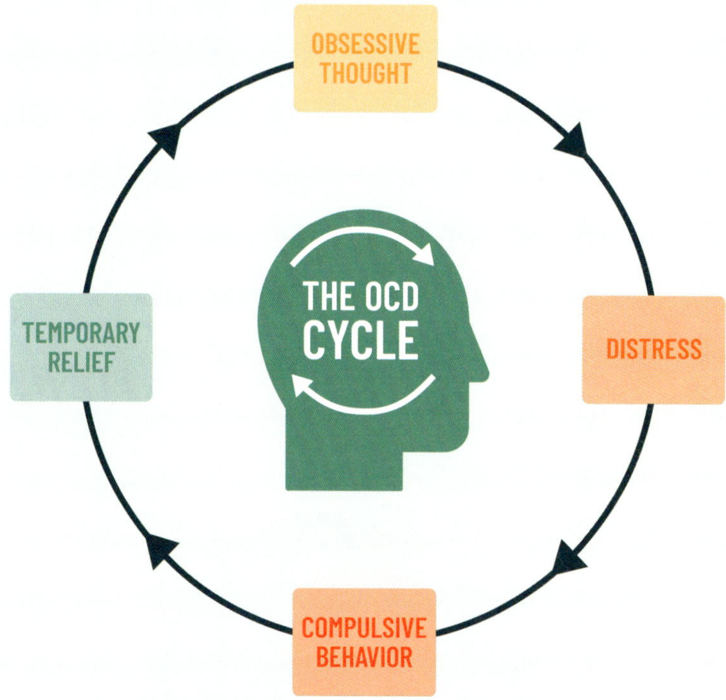

Source: Fjolla Arifi, "What Is the OCD Cycle? The Four Steps of OCD," NOCD, *November 27, 2024. www.treatmyocd.com.*

The OCD cycle feeds itself, which can make it difficult to break. However, specialized OCD treatment can disrupt the cycle and reduce OCD symptoms.

OCD happens in a cycle. It starts with an obsessive thought. The thought makes the person feel distress. The person completes a compulsive action to feel better. People with OCD may believe they can stop their obsessions if they complete the compulsions. But the thought eventually comes back. And the cycle starts again.

For example, a person with OCD might worry about getting sick from germs on their hands. They wash their hands as a compulsion. But then the worry comes back. They wash their hands again. These **rituals** can take a lot of time. They can get in the way of a person's daily life.

OBSESSIONS

Obsessions can cause people with OCD a lot of stress. People may feel ashamed and worried about their obsessive thoughts. Almost anything can become an obsession. But some obsessions are shared by many people with OCD.

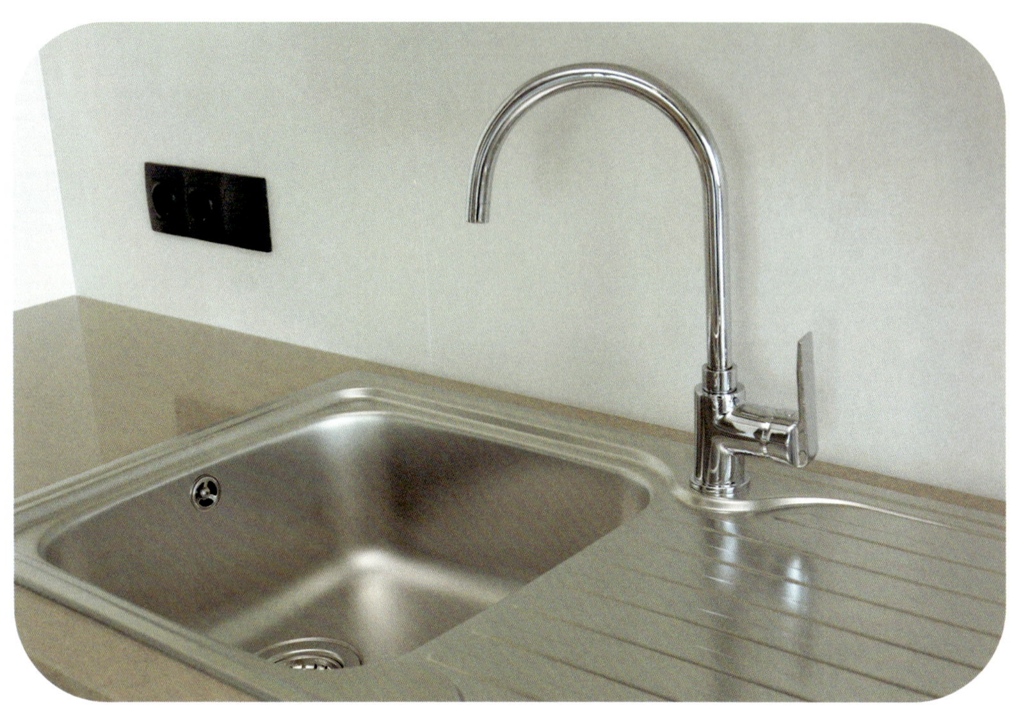

A person with OCD may consider kitchen sinks to be contaminated surfaces.

One common worry is **contamination**. People worry about touching things they believe to be unclean. These can include dirt and sticky things. They can also include surfaces that often have lots of germs. People may also worry about the possibility of getting sick.

Another common fear is people getting hurt. People with OCD may worry that someone else will be harmed. A teen with OCD might worry about their parents getting sick or dying. They may worry that something they do will hurt someone else. A person with OCD might repeatedly check to make sure the oven is turned off. They may worry about starting a fire that could hurt someone else.

Some people with OCD have obsessions about violence. They worry that they might harm themselves or someone else. They do not actually engage in violent behavior. But they cannot help fearing that they might.

Some people with OCD need things to be in a certain place or order. They may order things by color. Or they might need things to be arranged in straight lines. The wrong arrangement can cause distress.

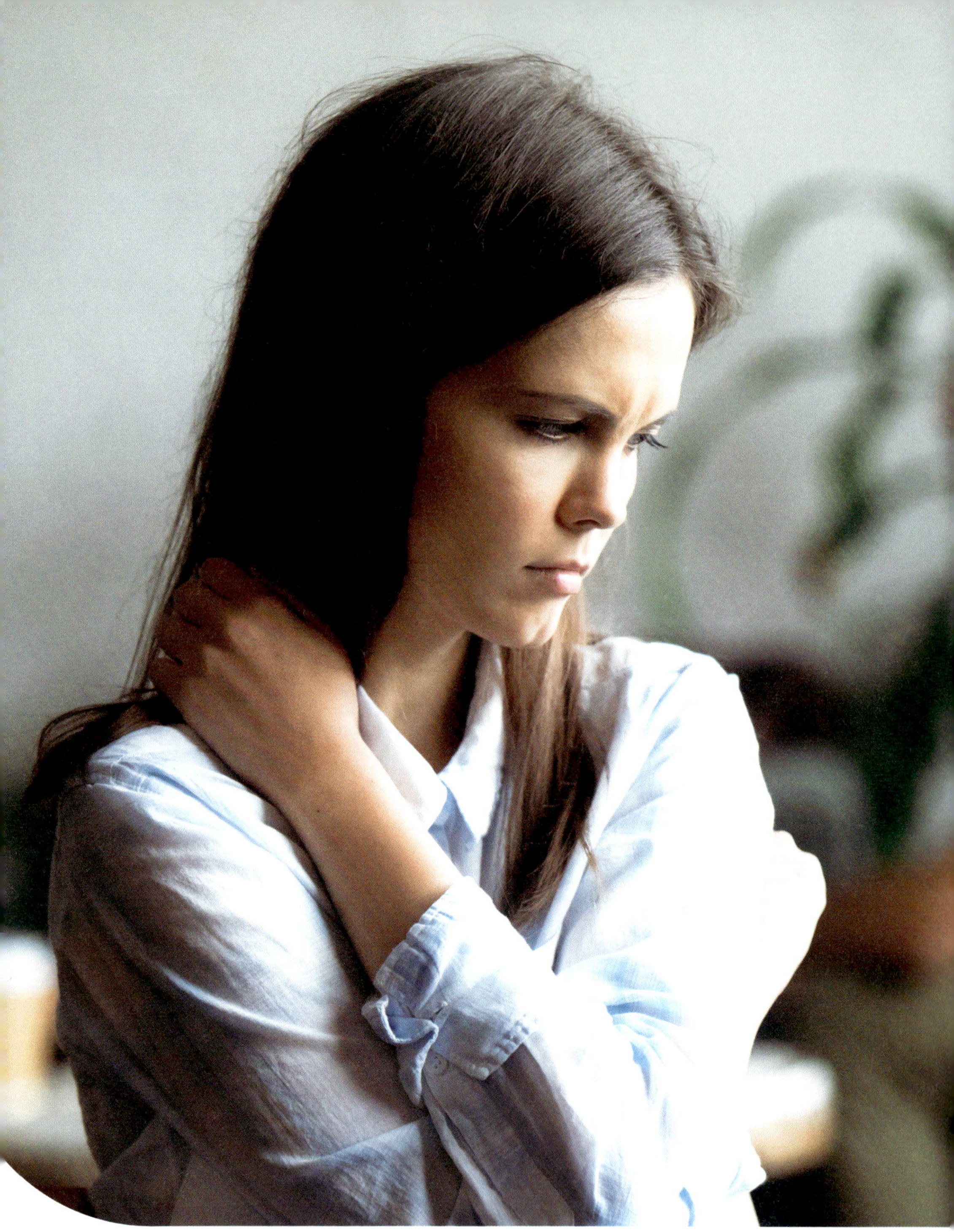

Teens with violence-related obsessions may isolate themselves out of fear of harming others.

People with OCD may also worry about misplacing or forgetting important items. They may have trouble deciding whether to keep or get rid of something.

Obsessions can be scary and tiring. They can cause physical symptoms. People with OCD might get stomachaches or headaches. Their disturbing thoughts can raise their heart rate. Their breathing may speed up as well.

People with OCD may understand that their obsessions are not realistic. They might know that their compulsions will not settle their worries. But they struggle to break the cycle anyway. Holden is a young person with OCD. He explains, "I know [my obsessions are] unbelievable . . . but [they are] just so real to me."[1]

COMPULSIONS

Compulsions bring temporary relief to people with OCD. But compulsions do not remove the original obsession. Engaging in compulsions actually makes obsessions more deeply rooted. This is why people with OCD typically repeat their compulsions.

Washing and cleaning are compulsions for some people with OCD. Some wash their hands over and over again. Others wash things a certain number of times or in a particular order. People may need to wash in a certain way in the shower. Or they may compulsively brush their teeth. Frequently cleaning the house or washing clothes can also be compulsions.

Checking is another compulsion. People might repeatedly check that the door is

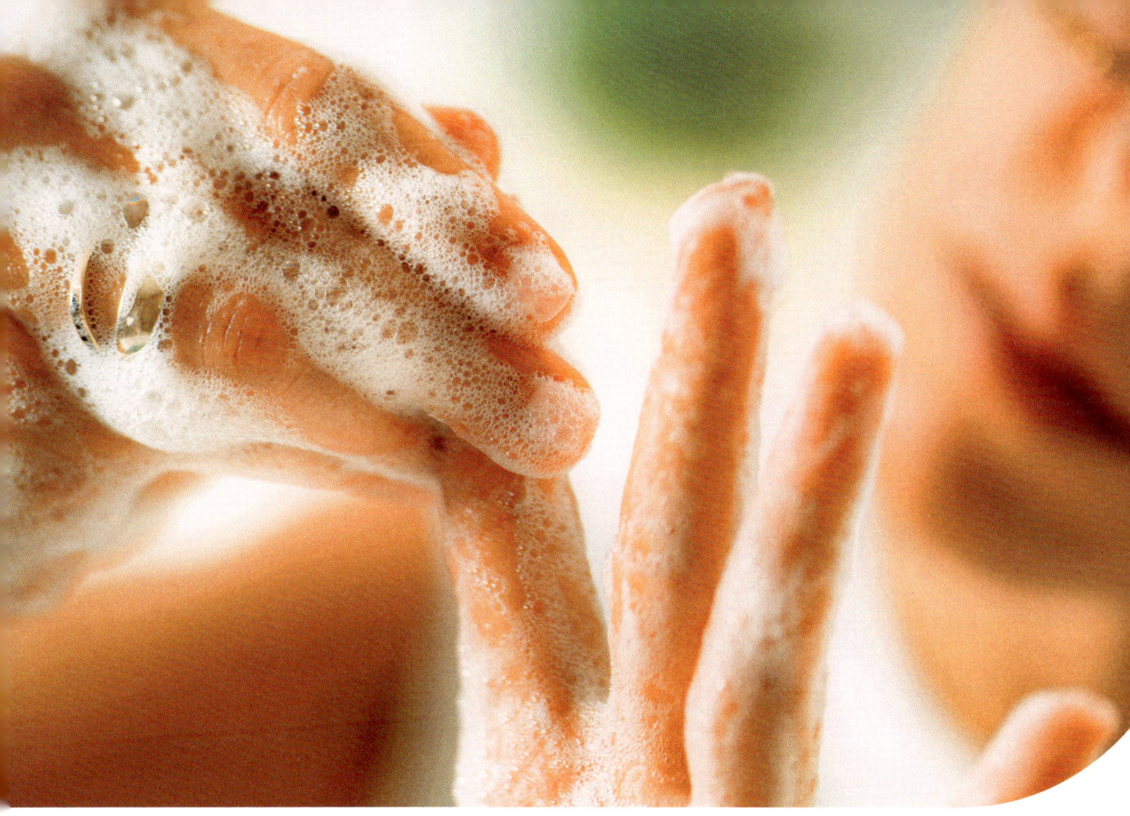

Ritual handwashing can be a symptom of OCD.

locked before leaving home. They might check that the stove is off. Teens with OCD might repeatedly check that they have packed an item in their backpack. And they might check that everyone is healthy before leaving home.

Counting things or actions can be compulsions. A person with OCD might need to turn the lights on and off four times before leaving a room. They may need to begin an activity again if they are interrupted.

STUDYING OCD

It is difficult to estimate how many people have OCD. This is because some people with OCD do not know they have it. Some estimates say that about one in

Mental Compulsions

Some compulsions are mental compulsions. These take the form of thoughts. Praying repetitively in one's head can be an example of a mental compulsion. Reviewing memories or past conversations can be mental compulsions too. Some people may only have mental compulsions. They might not recognize these thoughts as compulsions.

forty people will develop OCD in their lifetimes. People can develop the condition at any age. But it often starts within certain age ranges. The first range is between ages 7 and 12. The second range is between the late teens and about age 20.

OCD is a lifelong condition in most cases. Some people display their first OCD symptoms long before they are **diagnosed** with the condition. Obsessions and compulsions can come and go. And OCD can get worse when people are under more stress.

Scientists are studying OCD. They have learned that OCD does not have one simple cause. Instead, several risk factors likely come together to make a person more likely to develop OCD. One risk factor may be a

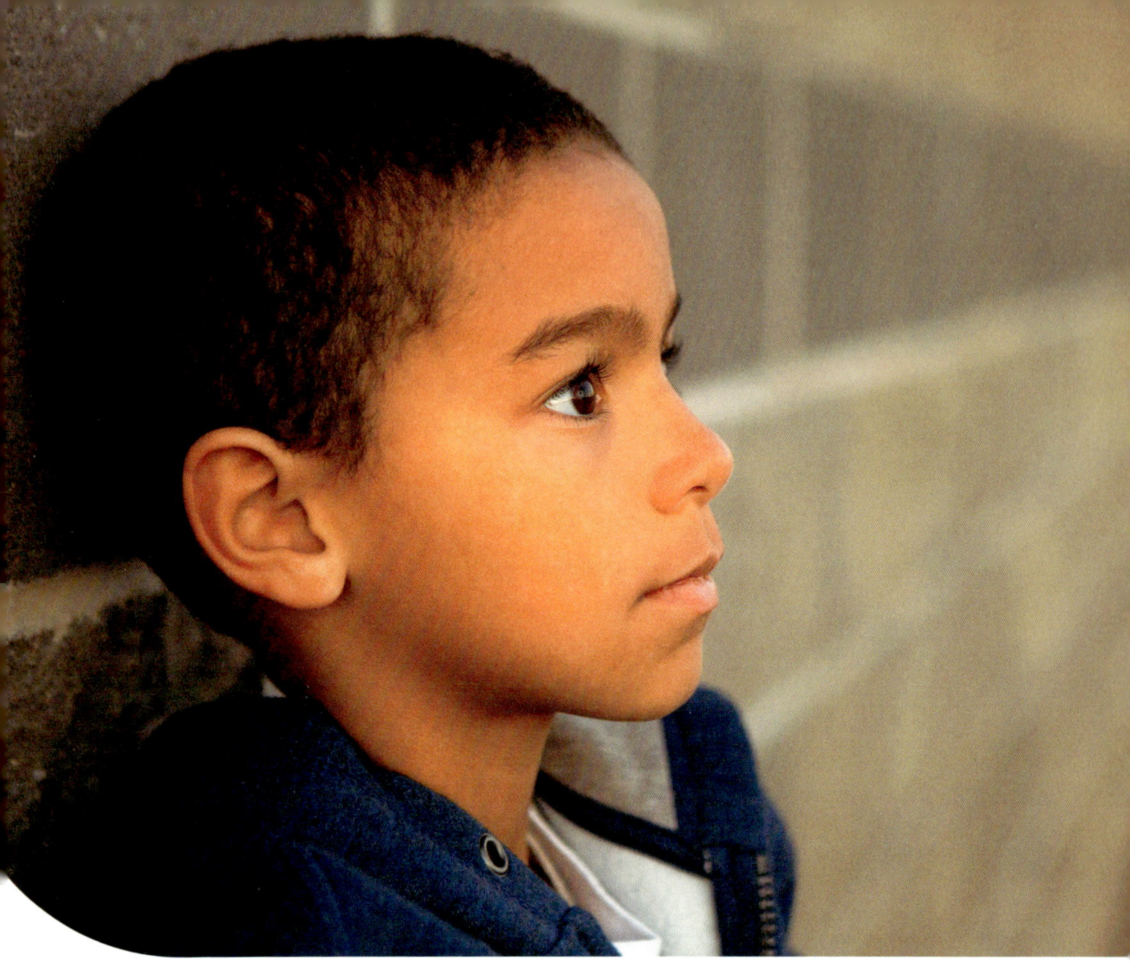

People with OCD may remember having preferences or habits as children that they later recognize to be OCD symptoms.

difference in brain structure. This difference may raise a person's risk of developing OCD. Another possible risk factor of OCD involves brain chemicals. The relationship between OCD and a brain chemical called **serotonin** has been studied. OCD may also be partly inherited. Children of parents with OCD are more likely to develop OCD themselves. This could mean that OCD risk can be passed on like traits such as hair color.

Obsessions and compulsions may be related to a person's culture. A person may have compulsions to pray. Events in the environment can also affect a person's OCD. The spread of a disease through a community can become part of a person's obsessions.

Environmental factors can also worsen a person's OCD symptoms. One of these factors is called accommodation. This is when people help a person with OCD perform their compulsions. Sometimes caregivers of a teen with OCD practice accommodation. They may do this because they want to relieve the teen's negative feelings. But accommodation can actually reinforce a teen's OCD. Treatment of a teen's OCD typically involves helping

It is natural for caregivers to want to comfort those in their care. But accommodating compulsions can have negative effects.

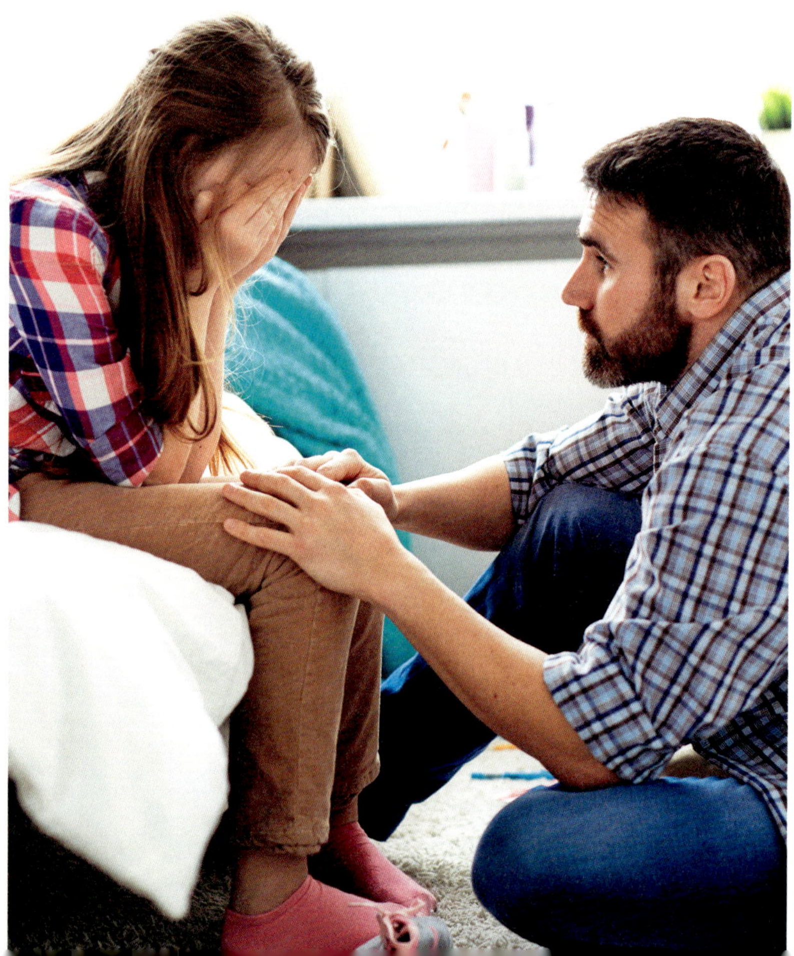

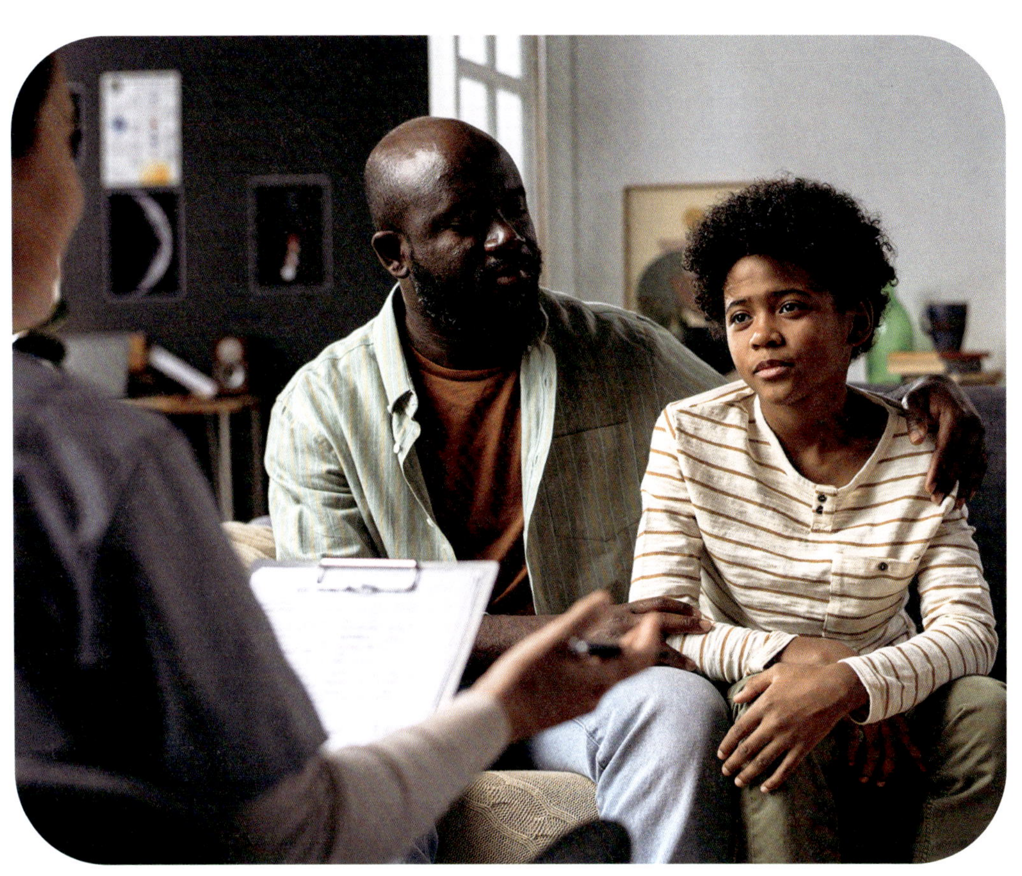

Limiting accommodation is a cooperative effort that can play a big role in a teen's treatment for OCD.

caregivers address accommodation. The teen, their caregivers, and their treatment providers work as a team to create a supportive environment and limit accommodation over time.

CHAPTER TWO

LIVING WITH OCD

Having OCD can get in the way of a teen's daily life. Their obsessions can feel overwhelming. And their compulsive rituals can take a lot of time. Teens with OCD may stop seeing friends. They may have trouble attending sport and club meetings. Staying home may feel more comfortable.

People are usually diagnosed with OCD when their obsessions or compulsions

OCD can cause significant distress and feelings of isolation in teens.

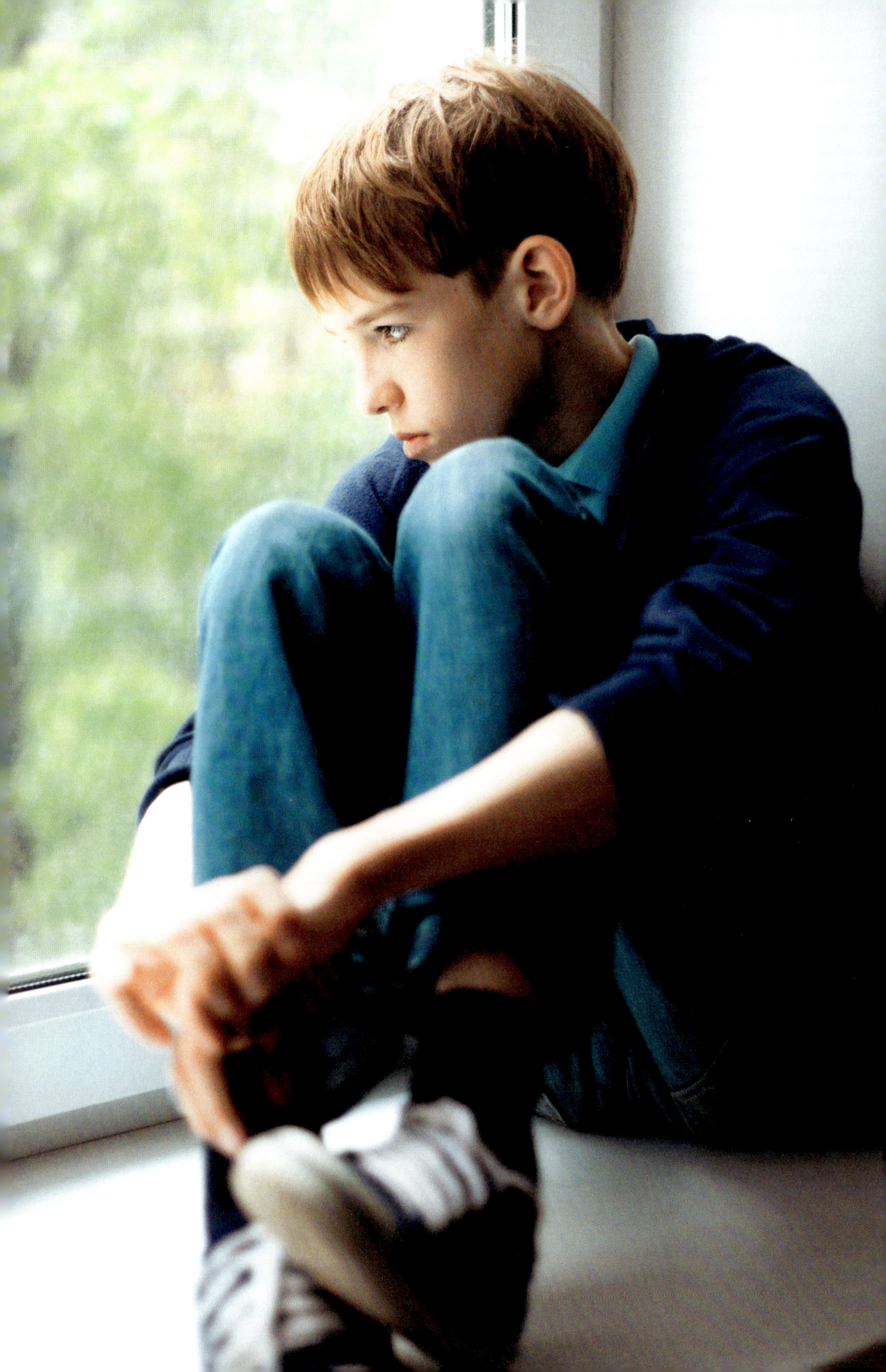

cause significant distress or get in the way of daily life. Georgina is a teen with OCD. She has a contamination obsession. Her compulsions have to do with cleaning and washing. She washes her body

A teen's OCD can cause them distress in their relationships with others.

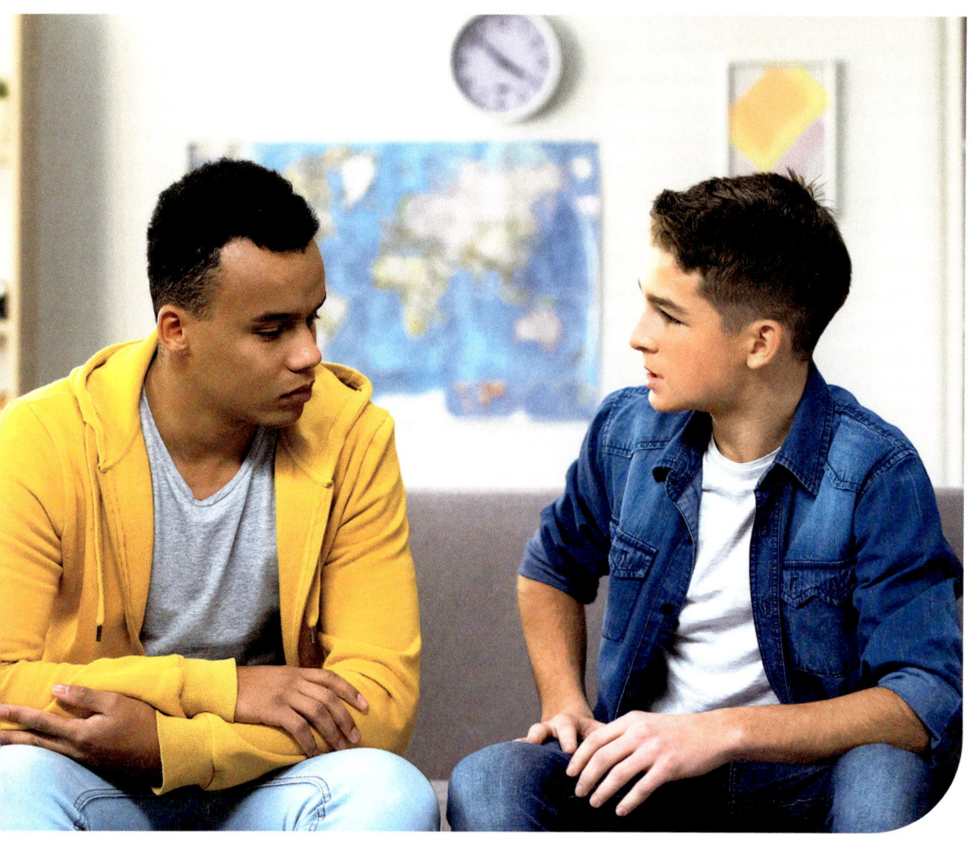

over and over again. She also cleans the surfaces in her home. When her condition is at its worst, her rituals take up to 10 hours a day. Sometimes she does not even stop to eat.

OCD AND OTHER PEOPLE

OCD can affect a teen's relationships with other people. A teen with OCD may have less time and energy for friendships. And sometimes a teen's relationships can become part of their OCD. A teen may worry that their friends do not really like them. This can become an obsession. One compulsion may be asking their friends for **reassurance**.

A teen's OCD can also involve their family. Stacy developed OCD when she was very young. Sometimes she asked her parents to accommodate her compulsions. She asked them to wash clean clothes when she thought they were dirty. She also worried that she had accidentally poisoned her loved ones. She would confess her fears to her parents for reassurance.

Stacy's OCD persisted during her teen years. The condition made her question what was real and what was imagined. She feared that she would no longer be able to tell whether her memories were real.

OCD AND SCHOOL

OCD can cause challenges for teens in school. A student's OCD can get in the way of their learning. And elements of the school

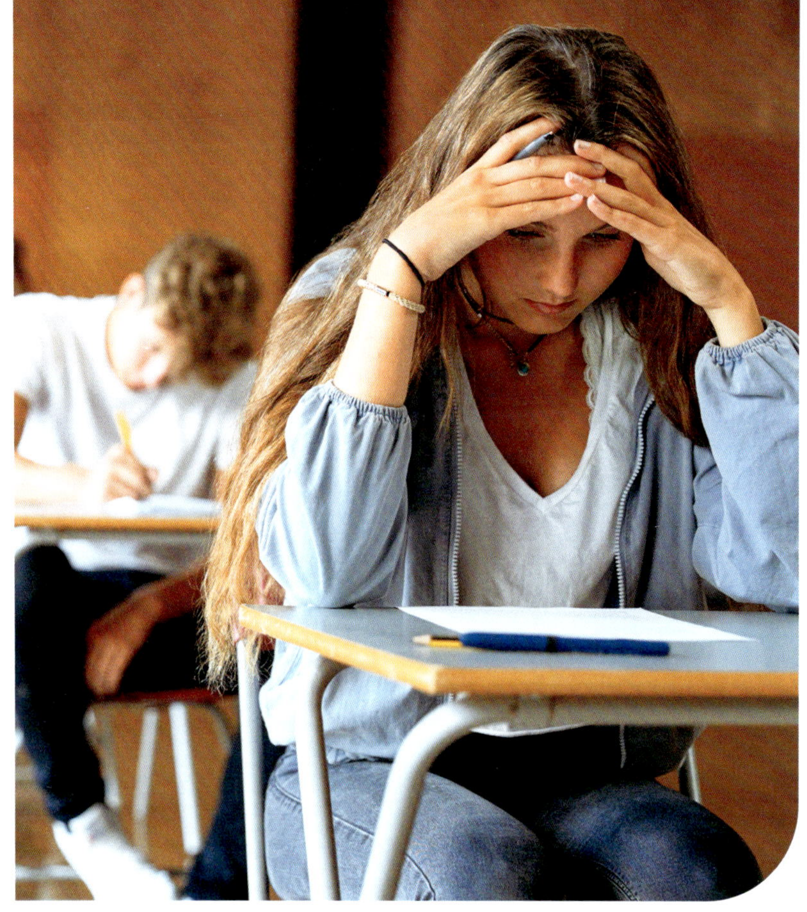

Symptoms that interfere with success at school may indicate that a teen has OCD.

environment can become part of the teen's OCD.

OCD can make it hard for teens to focus in class. Their obsessions may take their attention away from learning. Sixteen-year-old Rachel had contamination and harm obsessions. She worried that she was spreading a deadly virus to other people. Her compulsions included **excessive** washing rituals. Her OCD drew her attention away from school. Her parents and therapist decided to temporarily pull her out of school. She received intensive treatment for her OCD. Intensive treatment happens several days of the week for multiple hours. Once symptoms improve, students return to school.

Completing homework can be difficult for teens with OCD. Sometimes homework becomes part of the condition. Sean developed OCD as an early teen. He remembers, “I couldn’t touch paper to pencil without doing it 55 times before I wrote down a number for math homework.

It would take four hours, and I couldn't turn in my homework."[2]

HIDING THE CONDITION

Some teens may feel ashamed of their OCD. They may hide their symptoms from friends and family. This can make it harder to get help. Singer Camilla Cabello has had OCD since she was young. She used

David Beckham on OCD

Soccer star David Beckham talked about his OCD in a film about his life. He described his compulsions. He makes sure everything is neat at night. He checks that the lights are on the right settings. And he sets things around the house in straight lines or pairs.

to worry about what people would think if she talked about her condition. She says, "The little voice in my head was telling me that . . . people would think there was something wrong with me."[3]

Teens with OCD who feel ashamed of their obsessions may hide their distress.

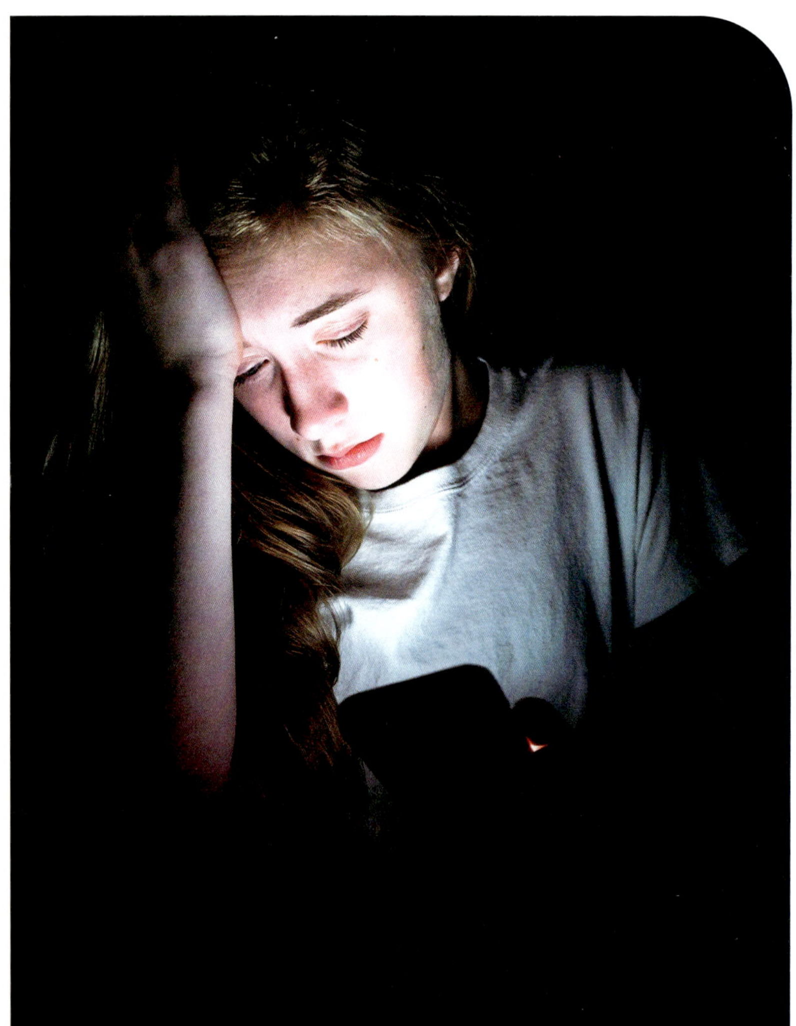

Obsessive thoughts can be scary. Teens with OCD may have thoughts about sex or violence. They may have thoughts about things they would never do in real life. This can cause them to stay away from other people. They fear they will do the things they are thinking about. Nicholas has OCD. He worked in a daycare as a teen. He began having obsessive thoughts about hurting the kids. The thoughts seemed so real to him. He felt like he needed to protect the kids from himself. This led him to quit his job. Nicholas never had and never would actually hurt anyone. But his OCD made him fear that he would.

Rebecca's OCD began in elementary school. She also had scary obsessions as a teen. She worried that people would

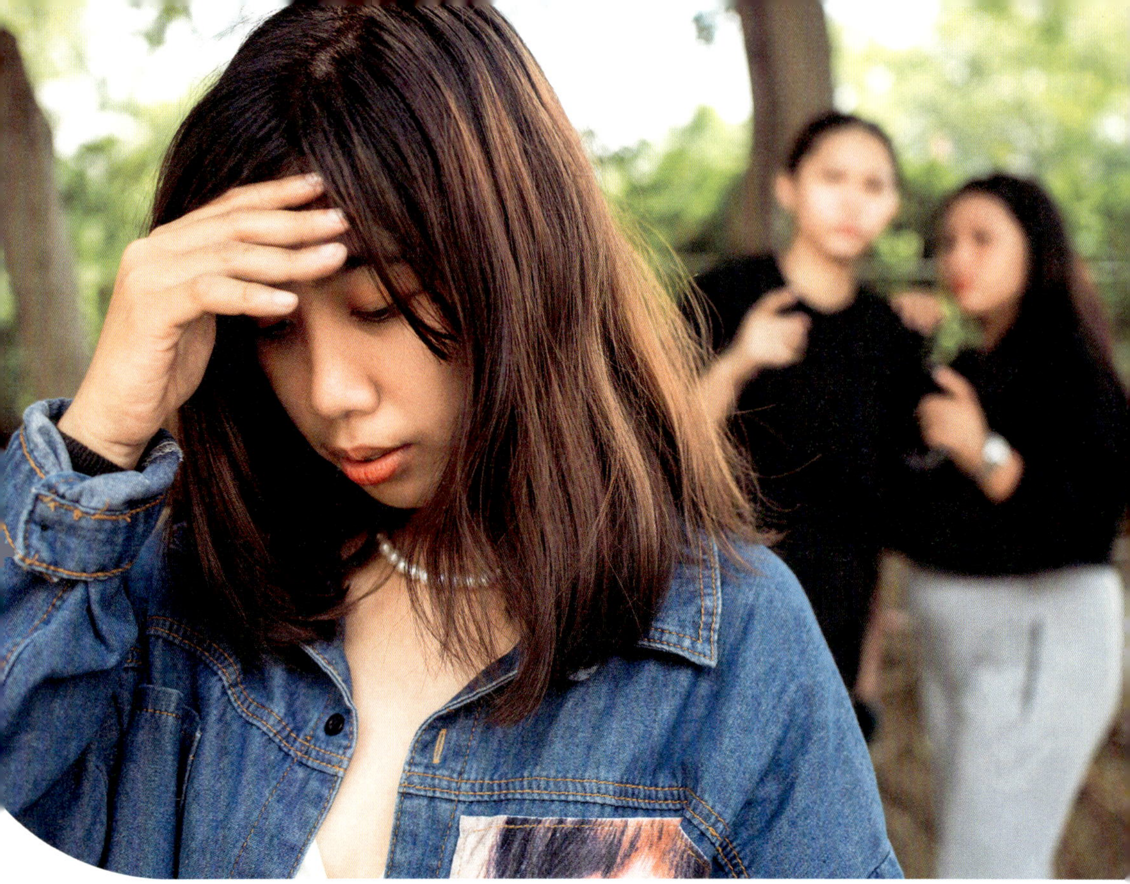

Studies have found that young people with OCD report higher rates of being bullied than young people without OCD.

find out. She says, "I used to think, 'Do people know what's going on in my brain? What if someone found out?' I wondered, 'Am I at risk for doing these things?'"[4]

Teens with OCD may feel ashamed about their compulsions as well as their obsessions. They might worry that people will think they are abnormal. So teens with OCD may try to hide their compulsions.

Jamal is a teen with OCD. He used to be an outgoing member of the rugby team. But his life changed when his contamination compulsions got worse. He became secretive. He quit rugby. And he started avoiding his family and friends. His parents noticed that he began to use more soap and toilet paper. They knew he was struggling with something serious.

Sam's OCD began when he was 7 years old. He developed many compulsions over time. He breathed on his hands. He counted when he got dressed. And he said repetitive prayers. Sam's compulsions made him feel embarrassed at school. Bullies sometimes targeted him.

FINDING HELP

Teens with OCD usually need mental health treatment to manage their symptoms. The first step is to find mental health professionals that are experts in treating OCD in kids and teens. A family doctor can refer the teen to an OCD professional. Teens and their families may also seek out a professional on their own. Professional organizations can help in this process. These organizations include the

Teens with concerns about OCD can talk with their doctors about getting tested for the condition.

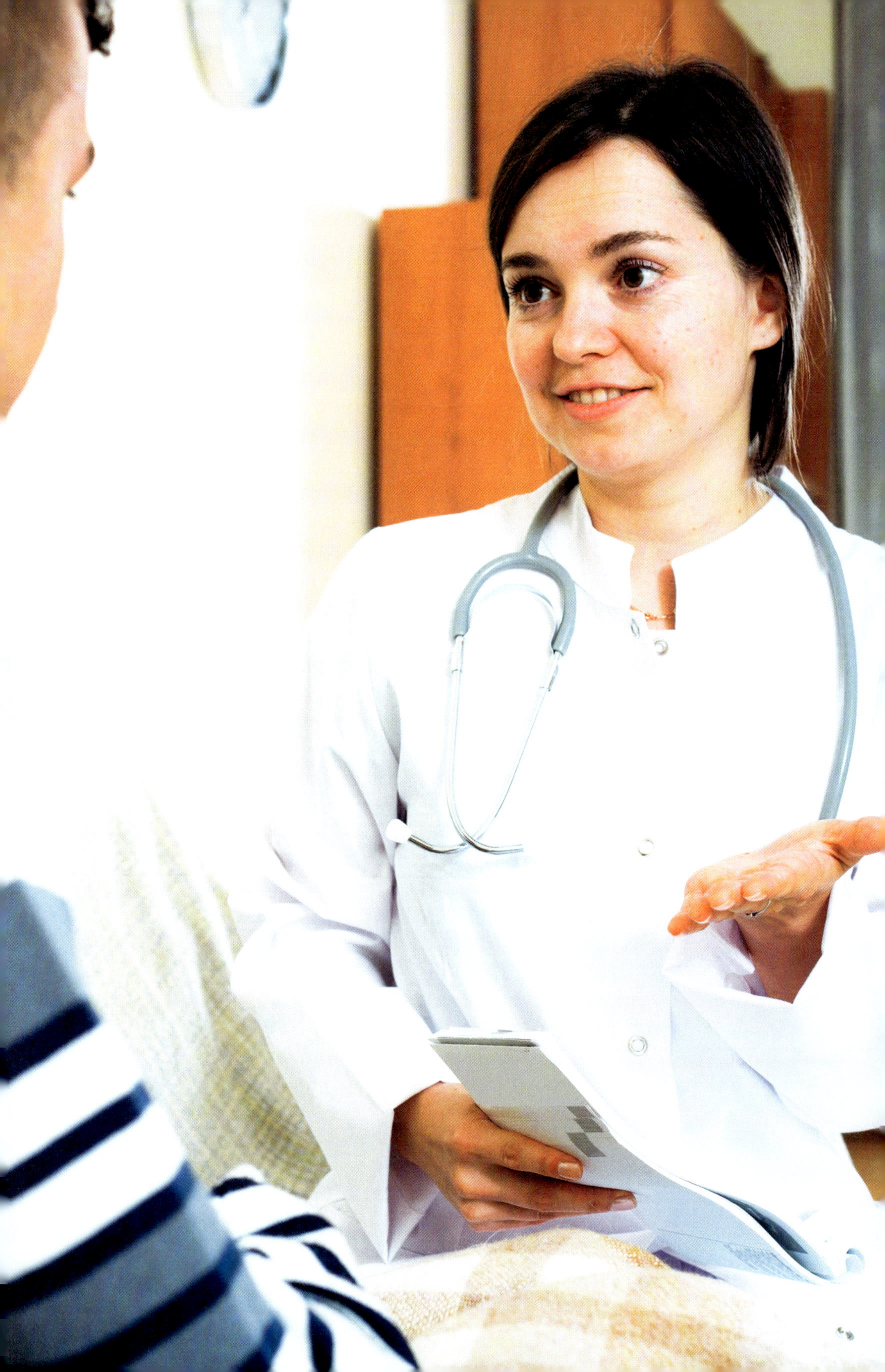

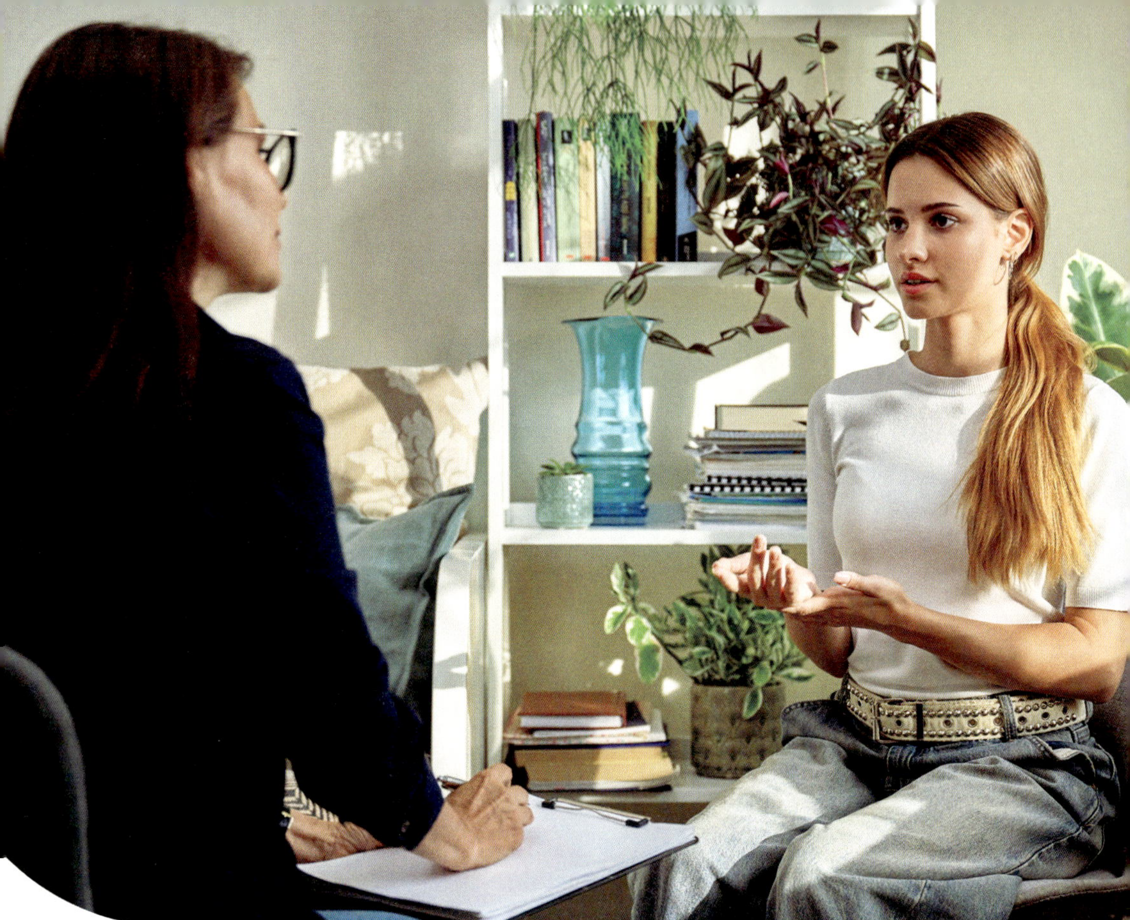

Not every kind of therapy is an appropriate treatment for OCD.

International OCD Foundation (IOCDF). They also include the Anxiety & Depression Association of America (ADAA).

There are two main treatments for OCD. They are therapy and medication. The combination of both treatments is more effective than either alone.

THERAPY

Therapy can be helpful for many mental health conditions. Patients typically meet their therapists for weekly sessions. There are different kinds of therapy. Some are suited to certain mental health conditions.

The most effective form of therapy for OCD is called exposure and response prevention (ERP). ERP seeks to help OCD patients break the cycle of obsessions and compulsions. It does this by slowly and safely exposing patients to what causes their distress. The patient and therapist work together to agree on an exposure plan. Exposures begin after teens learn lots of skills to help them handle distress. The patient is then urged not to engage in their compulsions. Over time, people learn

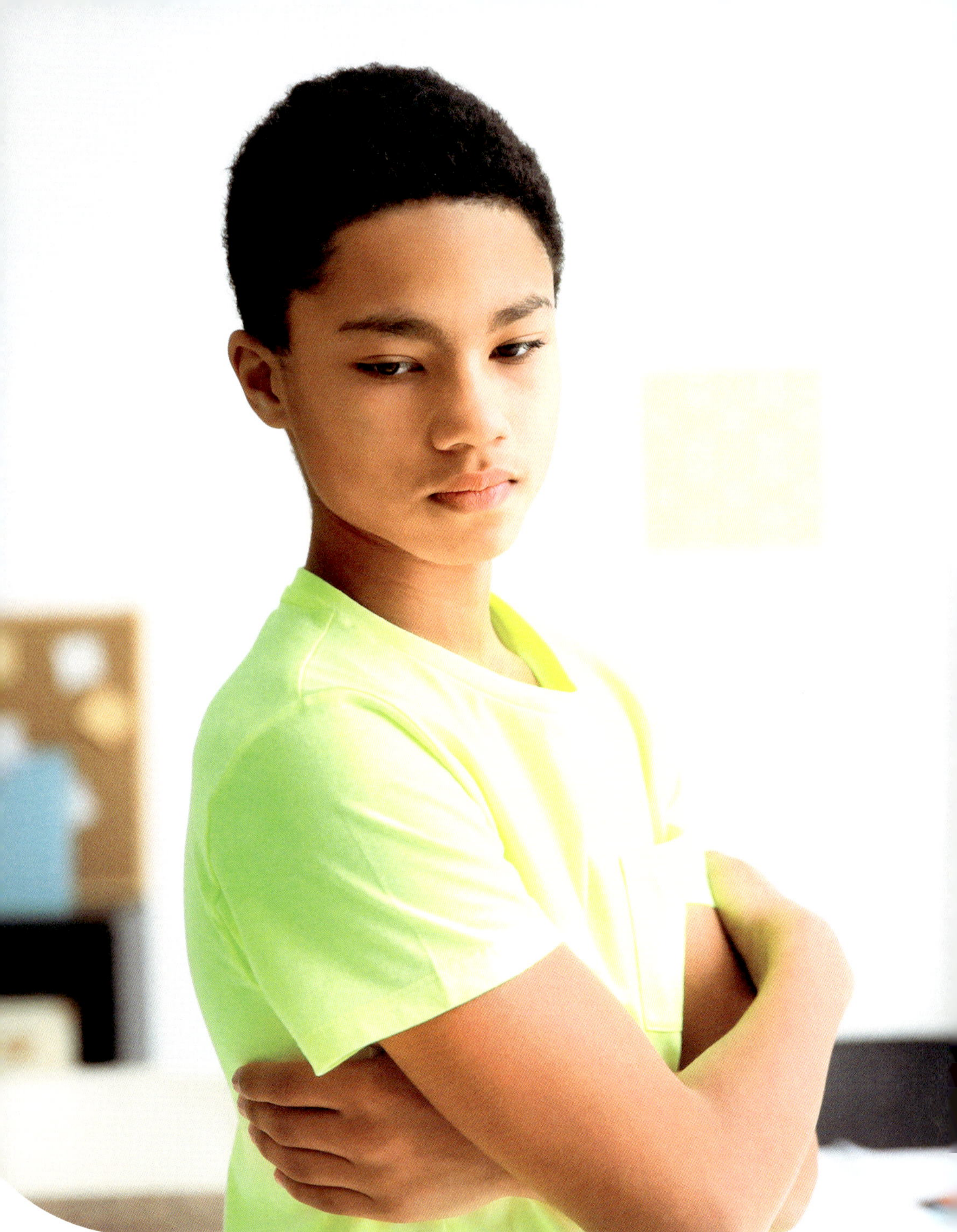

Exposure tasks can cause a lot of distress. That is why it is important for patients with OCD and their providers to agree on an exposure plan.

that they can tolerate the distress of the obsession without doing a compulsion.

Christine has OCD. Her obsessions have to do with germs. She uses ERP to face her fears. Her therapist gives her exposure tasks. They practice these tasks in therapy sessions at first. Then Christine starts to practice them at home. She started with easier things first. She put her backpack on her bed. This made her uncomfortable. She feared that her backpack was spreading germs to her bed. She wanted to remove it and wash her hands. But she sat with her feelings instead. She did not feel completely better at first. A single exposure session will not usually relieve a patient's negative feelings. But over weeks and months, ERP can lead to symptom relief.

Stacy learned that she had OCD at age 15. ERP gave her the tools to manage her symptoms. Now she is an OCD specialist. She works to help people with OCD take control of the condition. "Treatment is hard, living with OCD is harder, at some point you will need to choose your hard [option]," she says.[5]

MEDICATION

Antidepressants are the most common medications used to treat OCD.

These medications are not used to treat depression only. They are also used to treat other mental health conditions.

These medications affect the production and absorption of serotonin in the brain.

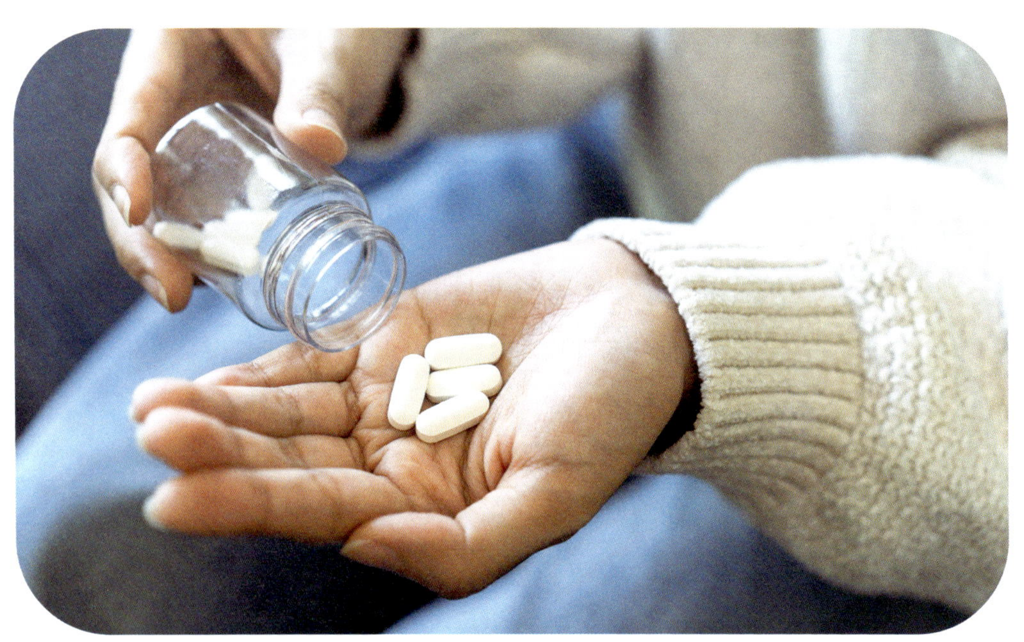

Antidepressants typically come in tablet or capsule form.

They have been shown to improve OCD symptoms for some patients.

Different people benefit from different amounts of medication. Professionals such as pediatricians and psychiatrists help patients find the dose that is best for them. OCD medication typically works slowly. It can take up to 12 weeks for it to have the intended effect at the right dose.

There are different kinds of antidepressants. Certain kinds may not work for a particular patient. Medication can also have negative side effects. Patients usually need to regularly check in with their doctors when first taking OCD medication. Doctors observe whether the medication is effective and if there are side effects.

Discontinuation Syndrome

People's bodies can get used to antidepressants over time. Suddenly stopping medication can cause symptoms. These include nausea and flu-like symptoms. This is called discontinuation syndrome. People taking antidepressants should talk to a doctor if they want to stop. The doctor can help the patient slowly reduce the amount of medication they take to avoid sickness.

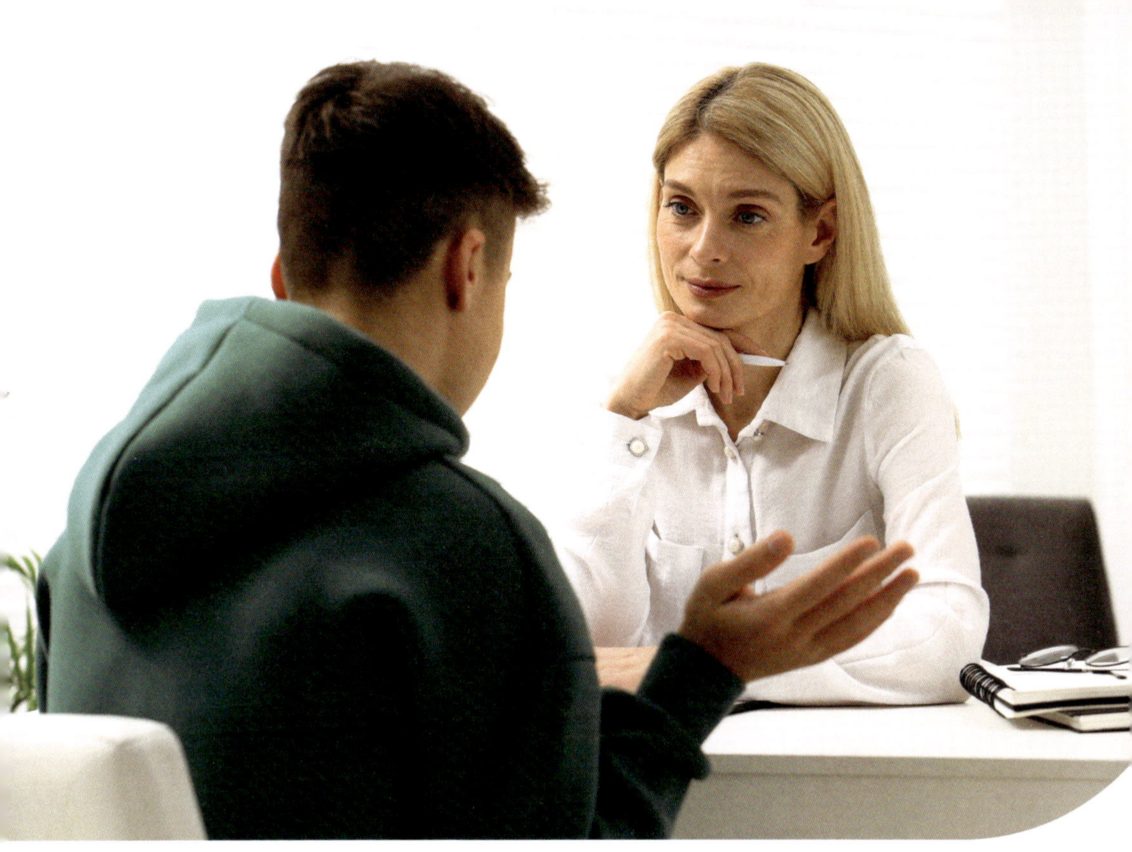

The IOCDF can help connect OCD patients with appropriate local treatment options.

Many people can successfully manage their OCD with medication and therapy. Georgina's OCD improved with therapy and medication. She has the tools she needs to deal with her obsessions. She still needs to use exposure to fight her symptoms. But she is more able than ever to live the life she wants to live.

OTHER TREATMENT OPTIONS

About 25 percent of people with severe OCD need more support than traditional therapy and medication. Some patients may need to go to therapy more than once

Loved ones of a teen with OCD can play a crucial role in the teen's treatment.

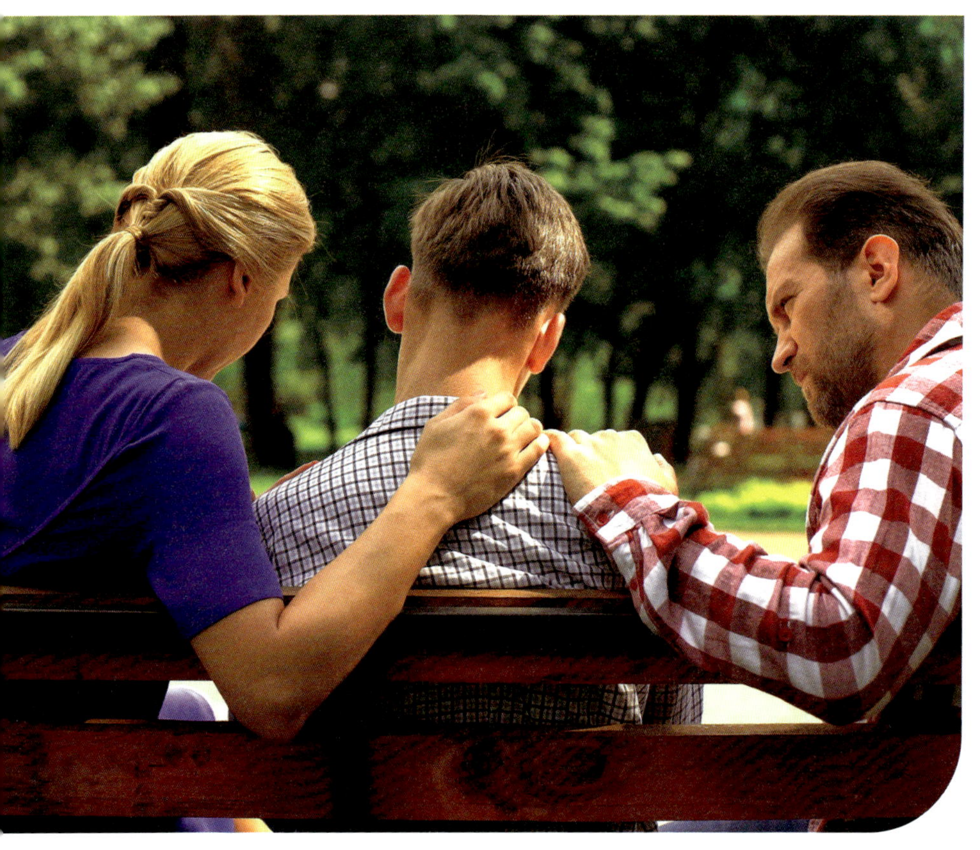

per week. Intensive outpatient programs can serve these patients. Patients in these programs attend treatment sessions for several days out of the week.

A teen with severe OCD may need to stay in a hospital or treatment center for **residential** therapy. A teen's caregiver may choose to place a teen in residential therapy. The teen might stay for weeks or months. Professionals at the treatment center help treat the teen's OCD using ERP and medication. ERP sessions may take place for several hours per day.

Robin was struggling for hours a day with her OCD. She went to a residential program. She stayed for 6 months. With the help of the program, Robin was able to manage her OCD with therapy.

She met other people who had OCD. "The [residential program] gave me a life, and I am forever grateful. . . . I don't know where I would be if I had not gone."[6]

SUPPORT FROM OTHERS

Teens with OCD do not have to go through treatment alone. Friends, family, and other loved ones can support teens with OCD. They can learn more about the condition. And they can listen as their loved one talks about their OCD. They can also help the teen recognize their compulsions.

One important way people can support a teen with OCD is being mindful about accommodation. People may try to help a teen with OCD feel better by encouraging their compulsions. A teen with OCD may ask a friend for reassurance. This may include asking the friend to tell them that they are not going to get sick. The friend may provide temporary relief by answering these questions. But it will not bring lasting improvement to OCD symptoms.

A supportive environment can help empower a teen during treatment for OCD.

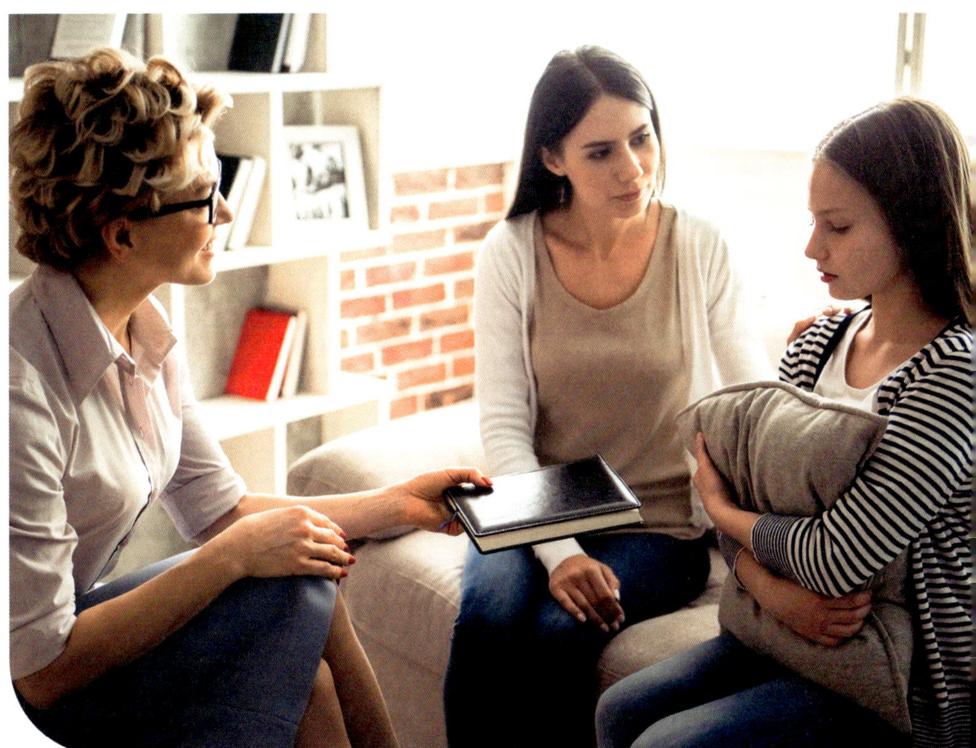

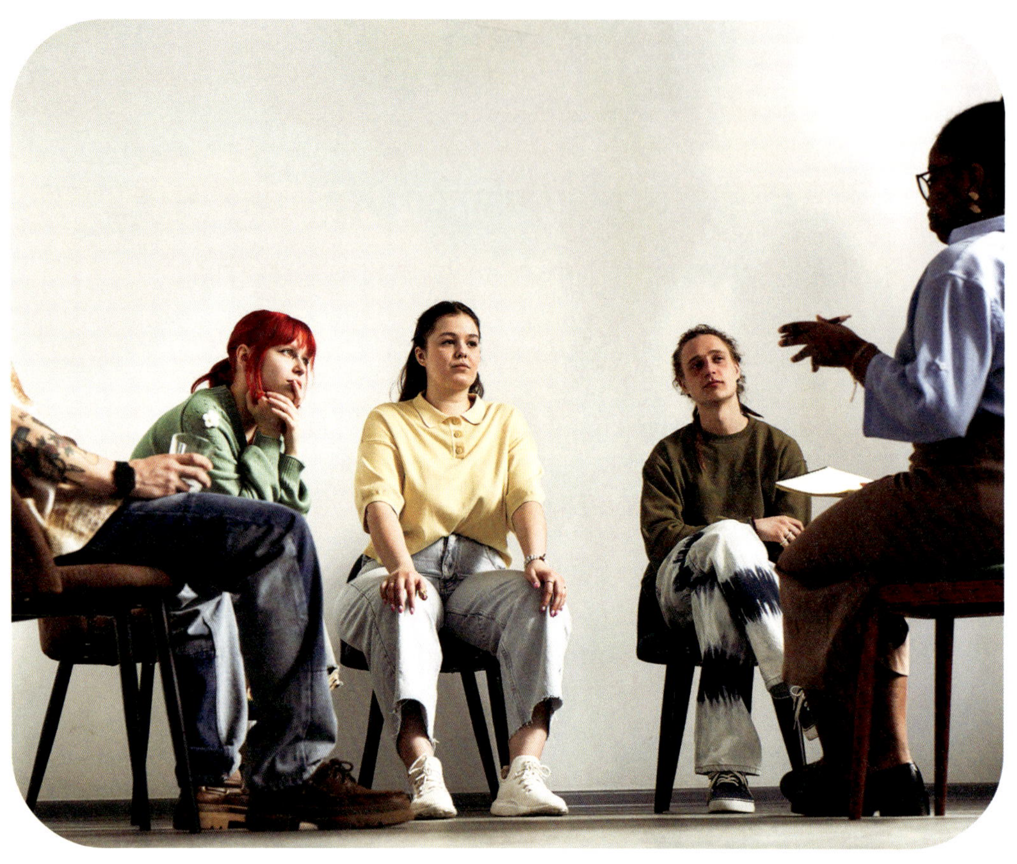

Support groups for OCD can serve as communities for people with the condition.

People can support teens with OCD by avoiding accommodation. A trained provider with experience treating OCD can help families find an approach that works. The provider may give families strategies for reducing accommodation slowly and with teens' agreement as part of ERP.

Peer groups and online groups can help teens meet other people who have OCD. These groups are not considered treatments. But meeting other people with OCD can help teens understand the condition. And helping others with their OCD can give teens a feeling of strength and hope. Victoria goes to a support group for her OCD in addition to her ERP therapy. She explains, "Supporting someone through their struggle can be a challenge, but it can also make you feel stronger and more accomplished. Everyone can benefit from peer support."[7]

Family members of a teen with OCD can talk to their teen's school. They can work with the school to make a plan for the teen. Nathaniel missed a lot of school because of his rituals and therapy. His school supported him and helped him get through the year. He was able to graduate.

Many teens with OCD have seen a reduction in their symptoms thanks to treatment.

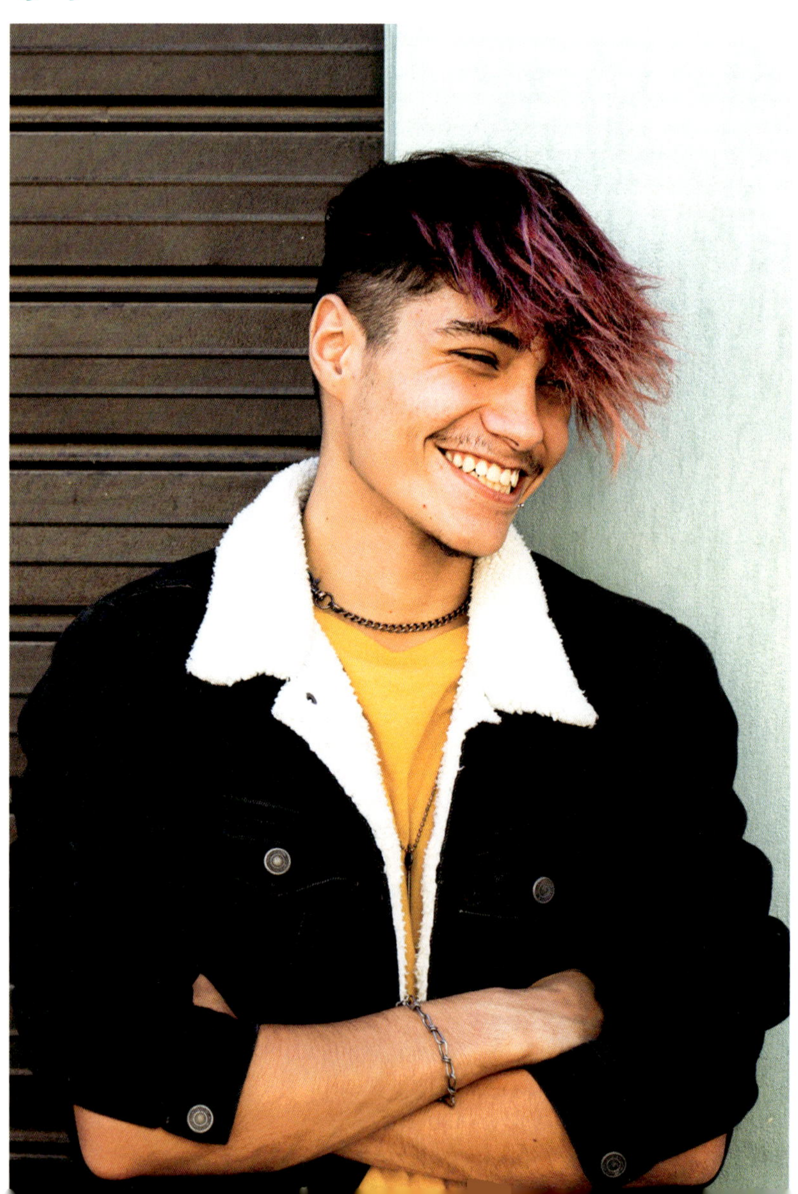

Now Nathaniel is a doctor who helps other people with OCD.

It can be stressful for a teen's family when their rituals take a lot of time. A teen with OCD can also get very upset. It can be hard to watch a family member struggle. Families can go to therapy together to deal with these feelings.

Mental health conditions such as OCD do not have cures. But treatment can help teens with OCD manage the condition. Treatment can give teens with OCD and their families the tools they need to take back control of their lives.

GLOSSARY

contamination

the state of being dirty or impure

diagnosed

identified as the cause of symptoms by a medical professional

excessive

going beyond what is necessary

medication

a substance used as a medical treatment

reassurance

statements that relieve someone's worries

residential

describing a place where people live

rituals

actions done in a precise way

serotonin

a chemical in the brain that performs many complicated roles

SOURCE NOTES

CHAPTER ONE: WHAT IS OCD?

1. Quoted in "What OCD Made Me Do: An UNSTUCK Extra Help Video," *YouTube*, uploaded by International OCD Foundation, February 25, 2019. www.youtube.com.

CHAPTER TWO: LIVING WITH OCD

2. Quoted in "I Lost 20 Years of My Life to a Lot of Pain Because I Was Scared to Talk," *Deconstructing Stigma*, n.d. https://deconstructingstigma.org.

3. Quoted in Michelle Pugle, "7 Celebrities with Obsessive-Compulsive Disorder," *Everyday Health*, August 8, 2022. www.everydayhealth.com.

4. Quoted in "I Knew I Was Struggling When I Became Afraid of My Own Thoughts," *Deconstructing Stigma*, n.d. https://deconstructingstigma.org.

CHAPTER THREE: FINDING HELP

5. Stacy Quick, "From Childhood Sufferer to OCD Specialist," *NOCD*, n.d. www.treatmyocd.com.

6. Quoted in "Patient Perspective: Reflections 20 Years After Seeking Treatment," *Mass General Brigham McLean*, June 21, 2020. www.mcleanhospital.org.

7. Victoria, "How Peer Support Changed My Life," *Mind*, October 14, 2021. www.mind.org.uk.

FOR FURTHER RESEARCH

BOOKS

Pan Cooke, *Puzzled: A Memoir About Growing Up With OCD*. Rocky Pond Books, 2024.

Where to Start: A Survival Guide to Anxiety, Depression, and Other Mental Health Challenges. Rocky Pond Books, 2023.

Philip Wolny, *Teen Guide: Helping Someone in Crisis*. BrightPoint Press, 2026.

INTERNET SOURCES

Jerry Bubrick, "First Person: A 13-Year-Old Learns to Fight OCD," *Child Mind Institute*, January 30, 2024. https://childmind.org.

Robert N. Kraft, "What's It Like to Be a Teen Living with OCD?" *Psychology Today*, March 7, 2023. www.psychologytoday.com.

"Obsessive-Compulsive Disorder," *Mayo Clinic*, December 21, 2023. www.mayoclinic.org.

WEBSITES

Anxiety & Depression Association of America
https://adaa.org

The Anxiety & Depression Association of America is an organization of mental health professionals who study and treat several mental health conditions, including OCD. Its website has information about OCD for patients.

Deconstructing Stigma
https://deconstructingstigma.org

Deconstructing Stigma is a campaign that aims to fight inaccurate and harmful attitudes about mental health conditions. Its website includes a page of stories about people who have OCD.

International OCD Foundation
https://iocdf.org

The International OCD Foundation provides information and resources about OCD. Its website has articles for those looking to learn more about the disorder.

INDEX

IMAGE CREDITS

Cover: © LP Design/Shutterstock Images
5: © StockPhotoDirectors/Shutterstock Images
7: © Steklo/Shutterstock Images
8: © DimaBerlin/Shutterstock Images
9: © Media_Photos/Shutterstock Images
10: © Darren Baker/Shutterstock Images
13: © carballo/Shutterstock Images
14: © elenabsl/Shutterstock Images
16: © Radovan1/Shutterstock Images
18: © fizkes/Shutterstock Images
21: © Microgen/Shutterstock Images
24: © Pixelheadphoto Digitalskillet/Shutterstock Images
26: © Pressmaster/Shutterstock Images
27: © Media_Photos/Shutterstock Images
29: © RimDream/Shutterstock Images
30: © Motortion Films/Shutterstock Images
33: © Monkey Business Images/Shutterstock Images
36: © mooremedia/Shutterstock Images
38: © MDV Edwards/Shutterstock Images
41: © BearFotos/Shutterstock Images
42: © VH-Studio/Shutterstock Images
44: © Africa Studio/Shutterstock Images
47: © Kmpzzz/Shutterstock Images
49: © New Africa/Shutterstock Images
50: © Motortion Films/Shutterstock Images
53: © George Rudy/Shutterstock Images
54: © SeventyFour/Shutterstock Images
56: © Simona Pilolla 2/Shutterstock Images

ABOUT THE AUTHOR

Diana Murrell is a teacher and writer in Ontario, Canada. She writes online lessons, educational video game scripts, magazine articles, and stories. She has also published educational books about technology, sports, extreme jobs, and United States monuments.